Nutrition

Why What You Eat Matters

By Luke Blackwell

Table of Content

Introduction

Welcome and thank you for buying this book, *"Nutrition: Why What You Eat Matters"*.

By downloading this book, you are now one step closer to the healthy lifestyle you have been dreaming of. This book contains almost all the information you need to know when it comes to eating better including what you should eat and what you should not since after all, YOU ARE WHAT YOU EAT!

Nutrition is a pretty broad subject but in reality, it is all about eating the correct foods which give your body all the nutrients it needs and in the correct proportions. This is the perfect way to ensure that your body has optimum functioning and more importantly, to ensure that you stay away from the ever common diet-related illnesses. With the correct information on how to keep your meals nutritious, you will now be well on your way to a positive lifestyle change whether you just want to improve your health or if you wish to get fit.

This book will therefore tackle concepts such as nutrition, seeking to understand what it is and the science behind it. The book will also cover what constitutes a nutritious meal covering the various nutrients needed by your body. This is not forgetting tips on how to eat right which will cover which foods should be avoided and more importantly, how you should go about in the preparation of your food. The book will also over the implications of nutrition to your health and also to your fitness journey. Finally, you will get to learn why nutrition is so important to observe.

By the end of this book, you can expect to have a more enlightened approach to your eating habits with enough knowledge on which foods to go for and which ones to avoid. Remember, balanced meals are the best way to incorporate nutrition to your feeding habits!

GET READY TO START YOUR HEALTHY FEEDING JOURNEY TODAY!

Chapter 1: **Nutrition: You Are What You Eat**

Eating healthy has over the recent years become a major concentration point and stress point for thousands of people across the world. Why is this so? It is the simple realization that you are what you eat! Therefore, some of the most common fatal illnesses like cancer, diabetes and hypertension are partly as a result of bad feeding habits. Moreover, more and more "healthy feeding" diets and meal plans are popping up on the internet every other day. Without a proper understanding of what nutrition entails, you may find yourself in a bottomless pile of diets. Whatever your reason to want to take up a healthier lifestyle, actually understanding about nutrition and why every bite you take counts is paramount.

With that in mind, this raises another question all together. How do you go about eating healthy? How do you observe the rules of nutrition? To get you started, let's first understand the concept of nutrition.

Understanding Nutrition

Nutrition has multiple scientific definitions. However, it is most synonymous with *Eating a Balanced Diet*. Our bodies need a large variety of foods to get the correct amounts of nutrients for optimum health. This means eating food which will provide your body with all the nutrients it needs from proteins, energy and essential fats to vitamins and minerals.

Nutrition can also be taken to refer to the Science explaining how nutrients and other food substances affect the body and its processes whether it is reproduction, health, growth or maintenance. Nutrition in this case therefore follows food from the moment it is ingested into the body then to its absorption, assimilation, catabolism and finally, excretion.

In reality, what constitutes observing the rules of nutrition is eating a balanced meal. This is however a very broad definition. To help guide you more, there are a few common rules to be observed when you are going healthy.

Cheat Sheet of Some Nutrition Rules

Nutrition Tip One: Eat Regularly. On a daily basis, nutritionists recommend having five to six meals, breakfast being the most important among them. You can opt for three big meals then two snack meals during the day. Ideally, have something small to munch on every 3-4 hours to ensure steady blood sugar levels. Staring your body may lead to your body adjusting to starvation conditions which causes it to store more food. This may lead to future diet-related illnesses and complications.

Nutrition Tip Two: Do not eat right before going to bed. Eat at least 3 hours prior to allow for digestion to take place before you retire to your bed.

Nutrition Tip Three: Always go natural! If you can eat straight out of your garden the better! Refined and processed foods mess with the purity of food whether it is through the addition of additives or the removal of fiber content in unrefined foods. This applies to everything. For sugar, opt for natural sweeteners like honey, sugarcane juice and maple syrup over refined sugar. Same case applies to fats and salts which should be kept at a minimum.

Nutrition Tip Four: What you drink can make all the difference. If you are a lover of soft drinks and specialty coffees then it is time you switched to water. Water is the purest drink to take with multiple nutrition benefits and best of all, water has no calories if you are looking to get fitter. You can supplement with natural fruit juice, milk, or unsweetened tea every once in a while.

Nutrition Tip Five: Balanced Meals plus Exercising. The secret to eating healthy is not just eating healthy foods but balanced out proportions of healthy foods which includes all the nutrients needed by the body. Moreover, the best way to supplement your meals is with a little physical activity. In addition to keeping you fit, this will help burn any extra foods leaving your organs strong and healthy!

Scientific Breakdown of Nutrition

When it comes to understanding the science behind nutrition, the first thing to take into consideration is nutrient requirements. Through years of research, nutritionists have determined the proportions of different nutrients that are required by the body every day for optimum functioning. This amount of each nutrient is what is known as the nutrient requirement.

Nutrient requirement is determined by a variety of factors such as age, gender, physical activity levels and health. For instance, women aged 17-35 need more iron in their diet as compared to men of the same age due to their menstrual cycle.

Since each nutrient has its specific use in the body, the amount needed for each varies. For example, nutrients needed in large quantities like carbohydrates and proteins are measured in grams while quantities needed in smaller proportions such as vitamins and minerals are measured in milligrams. To know the amount of nutrients you require, nutritionists and dieticians have set estimated amounts for different sets of individuals known as Dietary Reference Values or DRVs. Through these DRVs, you can now be able to determine the amount you need for each type of nutrient as will be discussed in chapter two.

The DRVs are divided into three population sets namely:

- **Boys and girls** (aged 0-3 months; 4-6 months; 7-9 months; 10-12 months; 1-3 years; 4-6 years; 7-10 years)
- **Females** (aged 11-14 years; 15-18 years; 19-50 years; 50+ years; pregnancy and breastfeeding)
- **Males** (aged 11-14 years; 15-18 years; 19-50 years; 50+ years)

In addition to that, there is also the RNI, Reference Nutrient Intake, which is the amount of a nutrient that is enough to make sure that the dietary needs of most people within the above named groups are met. By referring to the values of these two standards, you can have a guide to know how much your body needs and therefore know what portions are adequate! The values tend to change annually with additional research and information and they can be found online with a quick Google search.

Chapter 2: **What Constitutes a Nutritious Meal?**

For optimum health, having a nutritious meal is a must. What is a nutritious meal though? In simpler terms, a nutritious meal is one that is considered balanced, or rather one that has all the nutrients required by the body in the correct proportions.

Nutrients are largely divided into two:

- Macro-nutrients. These are needed by the body in large quantities. Under macronutrients we have carbohydrates, fats, water, fiber and proteins.
- Micro-nutrients. These are needed by the body in smaller quantities. Micronutrients most comprise of minerals and vitamins.

To best understand what our food should comprise of, it is best to analyze each nutrient and what benefits it has to the body.

Carbohydrates

Carbohydrates are arguably some of the most common types of food. Carbohydrates are best known for being sources of energy for the body. Contrary to popular belief, cutting out carbohydrates from your diet is not a way for you to eat healthier! Carbs have their importance and use to the body and they should therefore be part and parcel of your diet. Avoiding carbohydrates will cause your body to derive energy from proteins which out to be used for body building and repair purposes.

The only key is taking them in moderation. Under portions, this varies based on a number of factors namely age, gender, health conditions and so on. Nutritionists have estimated the recommended daily intake for men at 252g and for women at 198g daily.

Importance: Dietary energy is mostly derived from starch and sugars. Ideally, over half of the energy we need in our bodies should come from carbohydrates. Carbohydrates are also turned into glucose upon digestion which acts as fuel for body tissues.

Sources: Pasta, bread, rice, sugar, pastries and any other grain-based products.

Proteins

Proteins are some of the most popular foods! On digestion, proteins are broken down into amino acids which are then used for various body functions. Proteins sourced from animals contain the full range of essential amino acids as required by the body. Protein from plant sources however requires vegans and vegetarians to combine various legumes to get the full range of amino acids required by the body.

So how much protein is enough? Food specialists recommend taking 0.6g of protein per kilogram of your body weight on a daily basis. This is around 56g for men and 45g for women daily.

Importance: Proteins are essential for the growth and repair of body tissues and body muscles. Proteins can also be used for dietary energy purposes, being responsible for up to 15% of the body's energy needs.

Sources: Red meat, fish, chicken, eggs, milk and other dairy products, beans and legumes in general.

Fats and Oils

When it comes to fats and oils, this is in reference to essential fats which are required by the body in small amounts. Fats are mainly of two kids:

- Trans-fats or saturated fats – mainly from animal sources

- Essential fats or unsaturated fats – mainly from plant sources

Unsaturated fats are necessary for body function since they are broken down into fatty acids which are then used for various body functions. Fats contribute up to around 11% of food energy in the body.

Excessive ingestion of saturated fats or trans-fats may lead to serious health complications like hypertension and obesity. Therefore, it is no surprise that the recommended intake is around 11% daily for saturated fats. The key is therefore to reduce the amount of saturated fats in your meals. Go for skimmed milk, use less fat when cooking, avoid frying and bake or grill instead, go for lean meat for example skinless chicken and so on.

Importance: Fats and Oils provide the body with energy.

Sources: oily fish, omega-3 fatty acids, olive oil and fat spreads like butter, cheese and peanut butter.

Vitamins

Though they are required by the body in small proportions, vitamins are very essential to the body processes. Moreover, most vitamins are not produced by the body and therefore have to be ingested in food or as supplements. How much you should take varies with each type of vitamin, your age, health condition, and gender. To be on the safe side, ensure that each of your meals contains at least one of the vitamin-rich foods named below.

Vitamins include:

- Fat soluble vitamins – Vitamin A, D, E, K
- Water soluble vitamins – Vitamin B6, B12, C, Niacin, Riboflavin, Thiamin, and Folate.

Importance: Vitamins are needed mostly for development of strong bones and teeth, improved heart, brain and nervous system functioning and for thyroid function to regulate metabolism.

Sources: Dairy and dairy products, iodized salt, green leafy vegetables, carrots, liver, beans, fruits like oranges, cereal and soy products.

Minerals

Minerals are inorganic substances needed by the body in minimal quantities for various functions like formation of teeth, bones, tissues and other body fluids. Being that they are essential but required in small amounts, extra care has to be taken to ensure that the body gets enough of all the essential minerals. It is important to note that nutrients are absorbed faster and better by the body when taken as food as opposed to when taken as supplements. To ensure you reach your mineral limit, vary your diet to include various types of food such as fruits, vegetables, meat and some carbohydrates.

Examples of essential minerals are selenium, manganese, copper, fluoride, iodine, zinc, iron, potassium, sodium, magnesium, calcium, phosphorus and chromium among other trace elements.

Importance: Minerals are great for improving your overall body immunity, better bone formation and health and also for blood formation.

Sources: beans, fruits like figs and apricots, vegetables like kale and spinach, fish, red meat especially liver, fortified breakfast cereals, soy beans and dairy and dairy products.

Fiber

Dietary fiber or roughage refers to a carbohydrate that is not absorbed completely during digestion since it cannot be broken down by human digestive enzymes. Ideally, you ought to consume 18g of fiber every day. However, fiber is one of the most overlooked foods. Lack of fiber in your diet can lead to gut diseases like bowel cancer and constipation.

Importance: Fiber in your diet helps to reduce cholesterol and thus minimize risk of obesity and also reduce risk of type-2 diabetes.

Sources: Whole grain, bread, vegetables like beans and lentils, and fruits like figs, prunes and plums.

Water

The importance of water in your body is often underplayed. In actuality, the human body cannot go for over 3 days without water. Water makes up around 60% of your body weight. For proper body functioning, you need to take 6-7 glasses of water daily. This however also depends on your age, gender, health condition and levels of physical activity. Hydration is important for example before, during and after an exercise session.

Constant drinking of water is necessary to avoid dehydration which impairs your performance and physiological responses.

Importance: Water lubricates the eyes and joints in addition to being the main component of saliva. Water also helps to regulate body temperature while also helping in getting rid of waste. Finally, water is the medium in which almost all body functions and reactions take place.

Chapter 3: How to Eat Right

When it comes to eating and how to eat right, everyone has an opinion! However, how do you know what is right and accurate information and what is not? There are three basic standards when it comes to eating clean. These will offer a guide to the most recommended types of food to go for. Ideally, your meals should contain foods that are unprocessed, unrefined and containing unsaturated fats.

Processed and Unprocessed Foods
You have probably come across this debate once before. Today, there are multiple highly processed foods classified as 'organic', 'trans-fats free' and 'sodium-free' among other terms. To better understand this, let us define processed foods. These are foods whose natural form has been altered whether by adding additives or through other food processing processes.

The biggest challenge when it comes to such foods is the fact that processing goes hand in hand with addition of chemicals to natural food, either to improve the taste or the shelf life. Some processed foods are even completely manufactured in labs. You have no way to gauge whether the added chemicals are good for your health or harmful, making processed foods very dangerous! It is therefore recommended that you avoid them and opt for unprocessed, natural meals. Examples of such processed foods are instant oatmeal, mayonnaise, hot dogs and pasta sauce among other canned goods.

Highly processed foods are known to contain GMOs or Genetically Modified Organisms which lead to complications like cancer, obesity and infertility.

The key is therefore to go as natural as possible. Whatever foods you can find fresh, it is best to go for that option.

Saturated Fats and Unsaturated Fats

Fats are very crucial to your daily diet contrary to popular belief. The only trick however, is that you have to ensure you ingest healthy or unsaturated fats as opposed to unhealthy or saturated fats.

- Saturated fats are dangerous due to their high cholesterol content. They normally appear solid under room temperature. These fats can put you at risk of getting cardiovascular complications, hypertension or even obesity. Examples of saturated fats are meat fat, cheese, mayonnaise and butter.
- Unsaturated fats on the other hand improve your immunity, heart functioning and health in general. Examples include fish oil, canola oil, peanut butter, avocado oil, olive oil and so on.

Therefore, substitute your saturated fats with unsaturated fats to start clean living. A great example is using avocado on your toast as opposed to cheese.

Refined and Unrefined Foods

First and foremost, refining is when the exterior fibrous bran coating in grains is removed. This therefore reduces the amount of fiber in your food.

- Unrefined foods are the ideal foods. In addition to the high carbohydrate content, they also have high fiber content which is crucial when it comes to digestion and avoiding constipation and hemorrhoids. Examples include whole wheat, brown rice, amaranth, quinoa, millet and brown bread.
- Refined foods also have high carbohydrate content. They are however less healthy in comparison. They lead to excessive weight gain if taken in very large quantities and also diet-related health complications. Such foods include white rice and white bread.

The roughage in unrefined foods makes a whole lot of difference as you get started on your 'eating right' journey. Opt for whole bread and other pastries the next time you're going shopping!

Chapter 4: Food Preparation

Nutrition is determined by a numerous number of factors. Top among them is how your food is prepared and stored. The methods used for this should ensure that nutrients are preserved from heat, oxidation or leaching to avoid health complications arising from food. This therefore means that even after selecting the best and most nutritious foods for your meal, how you prepare them might end up making all the difference! Therefore, we will highlight some of the best ways to prepare your meal.

Cooked vs Raw Food

A quick search on the internet will reveal to you that how you prepare your food does matter! Today, more and more people actually believe that cooking tends to reduce the nutrient value of food and therefore, they opt for raw meals where possible for example with salads. Is there any truth in this concept?

Cooked vs Raw Food

A quick search on the internet will reveal to you that how you prepare your food does matter! Today, more and more people actually believe that cooking tends to reduce the nutrient value of food and therefore, they opt for raw meals where possible for example with salads. Is there any truth in this concept?

The reality of the matter is that this is all dependent on the type of food. Both raw and cooked foods have their own set of benefits. For maximum gain, you should strive to eat a variety of both kinds of food.

Raw foods mostly comprise of seeds and nuts, sprouted grains and fermented foods. A raw meal should comprise of at least 70% raw food. This can become tiring over time making this diet hard to sustain over time. Cooked food is known to have a better taste and in some instances, cooking brings out the nutrients in food as opposed to destroying the nutrients.

Raw food activists argue that cooking or even boiling food:

- Destroys enzymes in the food.

- Causes the loss of water-soluble vitamins.

Cooked food advocates on the other hand argue that:

- Cooked food is easier to chew and digest. This goes on to make the absorption of food nutrients much easier.
- Cooking helps to kill any harmful bacteria and pathogens in food especially for eggs, meat and dairy.
- Cooking makes antioxidants more available to your body than in raw foods.

The fact of the matter is that various foods require different methods of preparation. When cooking, however, it is important to observe simple rules such as using small amounts of fat. Foods can then be classified as:

1) Foods that are best eaten raw include garlic, onions, cabbage and broccoli.
2) Foods that are healthier when cooked include meat, poultry, fish, legumes, potatoes, carrots, tomatoes, spinach, mushrooms, and asparagus among others.

Vegetarians and Vegans

When it comes to food preparation, the biggest difference comes in if you opt for a vegan or vegetarian lifestyle. Despite being popular lifestyle choices today, most people cannot differentiate the two.

- Vegans avoid all animal products including meat, eggs, dairy, honey and gelatin. Moreover, they will also avoid clothes made from animal skin and any products tested on animals. Veganism is mostly associated with a political statement for example in regards to animal rights and environmental preservation.
- Vegetarians on the other hand mostly stay away from meat and meat products. They may however eat other animal products like eggs, honey and dairy.

As a vegan or vegetarian, the key is to substitute your animal based foods with their equivalent in plant based foods. This may be harder since for plant based foods, you will have to combine a number of foods to get the maximum nutrient requirements as needed by your body. Keen attention should be paid especially to omega-3 fatty acids, calcium, iron, protein, vitamins D and B12.

Food preparation for vegan and vegetarian diets is much simpler since it tends to contain more natural foods and thus less cooking is required. However, where cooking is needed, it is important to ensure that minimal amounts of oil are used and the oil should ideally be vegetable oil.

If you are looking to have healthier and more nutritious meals, this is a way to go. Vegan and vegetarian diets pay close attention to nutrient content and all while cutting down potentially harmful food sources.

Here is a list of some of the best food substitutes for vegan and vegetarian diets:

Protein Substitutes

Since meat and meat products take the biggest hits, they can be substituted with plant-based options like:

- Soy foods such as tempeh, tofu, soy milk and edamame.
- Legumes including peas, beans, lentils and hummus.
- Nuts and nut butters like almond butter, peanut butter and sunflower seed butter.
- Meat substitutes such as veggie burgers.

Carbohydrates Substitutes

Vegan and vegetarian diets employ a lot of whole food substitutes high in fiber such as bulgur, tortillas, whole wheat bread, brown rice, pasta, oats and quinoa.

Fats and Oils Substitutes

These dietary options cut down on trans-fats and cholesterol. Great substitute sources for fats therefore are avocados, nut butters like peanut butter and nuts. You can also opt for supplements such as omega-3 oil supplements.

Minerals and Vitamins Substitutes

These are some of the harder nutrients to achieve. This is because meat and dairy products have a high, wholesome nutrient value content for vitamins and minerals as opposed to vegetable sources.

Mineral substitutes include zinc which can be found in legumes, nuts, breakfast cereals, soy foods, and whole grains, iron which is found in tofu, green leafy vegetables, soy beans, dried fruits likes prunes and apricots and beans.

Vitamins on the other hand may require you to take supplements for example for Vitamin B12. Other natural sources may include cereal, yeast flakes and soy milk. For omega-3, natural sources include canola beans, flaxseeds and tofu.

For iodine, using iodized salt is the best way to go. Vitamin D can be obtained naturally from the sun and also through foods like orange juice and soy milk and its products.

Chapter 5: Nutrition and Health

Having established that we are basically what we eat, then this simply means that bad eating habits are most likely to cause health complications and long term illnesses. The role that nutrition plays when it comes to health is very simple but crucial, if you want a healthy body, you must eat healthy. You must therefore avoid foods that are considered harmful and unhealthy, particularly foods which contain very high levels of sugar, salt or fats.

A change in feeding habits can lead to very big changes in your life, starting from better overall health due to improved immunity levels.

Diet-related Diseases

To best understand the implications diet and nutrition has over your health, we can take a look at some of the most common diet related conditions that crop up due lack of nutritious meals. Diet-associated illnesses are almost always fatal and once you contract the disease, the condition will require constant management where you will have to do a complete overhaul of your lifestyle and feeding habits.

Some of the major diseases associated with nutrition include; dental caries, osteoporosis, Type 2 diabetes, obesity, hypertension, stroke, coronary heart disease, dementia, gall bladder disease, some types of cancer, atherosclerosis and nutritional anemia.

Type 2 Diabetes

Contrary to popular belief, diabetes is not as a result of ingestion of too much sugar but as a result of continuous ingestion of high-fat and high-calorie foods. Over time, your body cells become resistant to insulin and making it almost impossible for glucose to enter the cells. All this excess glucose in the blood means that your blood sugar levels will be very high. This results in diabetes. Over time, other complications may arise such as heart failure, kidney failure, strokes, blindness, damage of blood vessels and even loss of limbs.

Prevention of diabetes is pretty simple. With a lifestyle change and eating balanced and nutritious meals, you will have nothing to worry about. Nutrition is all about eating the correct proportions of all nutrients needed by the body.

Obesity

A lifetime of living on junk food and foods high in trans-fats is a sure way to become obese. Obesity can however in some cases be a genetic condition. However, whatever the case, eating excess fats and carbohydrates is a major cause. During digestion, carbohydrates and fats are turned into glucose which is then absorbed by the body cells. Excessive amounts of glucose in the body are usually turned into fat and stored in the body for future use. This is where obesity originates from.

These excess fats normally gather around the heart and arteries and they may over time clog the arteries leading to cardiovascular complications such as heart failure, coronary heart disease or stroke. Ensure you eat just enough amounts of fats, oils and carbohydrates as recommended daily for your body.

Dental Caries

This is a condition where the teeth are gradually destroyed by acids from the bacteria acting on sugars and other fermenting carbohydrates on the surface of the teeth.

Teeth are very important but sensitive at the same time. Whatever you are eating, you have to take extra care of your teeth and gums by brushing and flossing regularly and also using the right kind of toothbrush and toothpaste for your teeth.

If you have a sweet tooth then you better watch out for dental caries. Eating foods containing extremely high levels of sugar every day is a recipe for disaster starting from issues like loss of teeth, tooth sensitivity, cavities, plaque and tooth decay. Ensure that you brush your teeth every day before going to bed so that bacteria does not have all night to destroy your teeth!

Nutritional Anemia

As explained earlier, all nutrients are required by the body to function properly whether in minimal or large amounts. Failure to supply your body with all nutrients may lead to some conditions like anemia as a result. Anemia is a sign of reduced red blood cells count which in turn results from poor diet and a deficiency of iron, vitamin B12 and folate.

To treat this, you have to increase your intake of iron-rich foods like meat, poultry, fortified cereal, eggs, and green leafy vegetables.

Hypertension

Hypertension is one of the most common illnesses in the world today. It is characterized by increased pressure in the blood vessels and heart. Also known as high blood pressure, this dietary illness is as a result of continuous ingestion of foods with high fat and salt content and also continuous abuse of alcohol and tobacco. Therefore, by cutting down junk food, trans-fats and alcohol, you stand a better chance of avoiding this condition.

Cut down on table salt and limit the amount of oil you use when cooking. These are some of the few dietary cut backs that will help you be well on your way to a healthier lifestyle.

Cancer

In multiple cancer cases, food and nutrition has been found to be a major contributor. This is particularly for forms of cancer affecting the stomach, blood, pancrease, mouth, liver and other parts of the digestive system.

Where does this cancer originate from? Research has found that highly processed foods can be a source of cancer. Too many chemicals in your food may prove harmful over long periods of use. A good example is mercury which was found to be in high content in a number of canned sea food. Prolonged eating of the food ended up being fatal. The best way to stay safe is to stick to natural and whole foods as much as possible.

Moreover, further studies have shown that fiber-rich foods are best for reducing chances of getting bowel cancer.

Chapter 6: Nutrition and Fitness

If the reason behind you wanting to eat better is to cut down the extra pounds and get fitter, then this is the chapter for you! The role that nutrition plays in getting fit is unparalleled. Actually if you wish to cut down the fat and build more muscle, the exercise bit accounts for just 20% while your nutrition accounts for up to 80%. Therefore, if you are hitting the gym often but continue to eat badly, you might end up not seeing any changes!

To fully understand the role nutrition plays when it comes to fitness, we will analyze each nutrient and its relevance to fitness.

Carbohydrates

As discussed earlier, carbohydrates provide the body most of its energy. Energy is essential when it comes to any physical activity and particularly for intense ones like working out at the gym be it cardio exercises or lifting weights.

Another important factor associated with carbohydrates is portion size. Eating carbs in excess can be problematic to your fitness. Excess glucose is turned into fat and stored in the body leading to conditions like obesity in the long run. Therefore, the secret is to stay away from junk and other harmful carbohydrates and stick to essential carbs for maximum energy for example pasta, rice, whole wheat and so on. You can also take a bit of glucose powder for an energy boost when you are doing highly intense activities.

Proteins

If you are looking to build your body and muscle mass, then proteins should be a key component in your diet. Proteins are essential for the growth and repair of body tissues and muscles. That is why body builders take protein shakes before intense weight exercises. Protein can also be turned into energy which is essential for high physical activity.

Therefore, beef up your protein intake with more red meat, poultry, fish, dairy and dairy products. However, remember that these foods also contain fats and if taken in huge amounts, they may end up causing weight gain.

Fats and Oils

Essential fats and oils are also very crucial when it comes to fitness. First, they are a source of energy for the body. Second, oils also contain minerals that strengthen your bones. Care has to be taken however to ensure that mostly unsaturated fats are taken and in minimal proportions. Eating cheese with every meal throughout the week may lead to weight gain as opposed to increasing your energy levels.

Vitamins and Minerals

Vitamins and minerals are essential for stronger bones and teeth and also for the better functioning of the brain and heart. With long cardio sessions at the gym, your heart functioning has to be optimum to avoid complications such as strokes or heart attacks. Athletes and other sportspersons can attest to the importance of supplements to their overall performance on the track, field or court. However, remember that it is recommended that you take your nutrients as food as opposed to supplements for faster absorption.

Water

Hydrating while working out is the law! In fact, you ought to drink water before, during and after your workout session. For days with high physical activity, drink 10 or more glasses of water to avoid dehydration which can cause brain complications over time. Water lubricates your joints which is very important as you are pursing fitness. Remember, water is life!

NUTRITION TIP: Simply changing your lifestyle and diet by paying attention to nutritional requirements is enough to help you reach your fitness goals.

Coupled with regular physical activity, you can expect to a healthier and leaner body in no time.

Chapter 7: **Why You Should Observe Nutrition**

All through the book, we have covered multiple importance of Nutrition. There are however some major reasons why proper nutrition should be top on your list.

Here are some of these reasons:

- **Improved Overall Health.**
  By paying keen attention to your what you eat and particularly the nutrient value on your plate, you can expect to have a better immune system and better health overall. Moreover, watching what you eat is a sure way to curb illnesses that are diet-related such as type 2 diabetes, heart diseases and high blood pressure.
- **Increased Energy Levels.**
  As seen in Chapter 2, observing the proper proportions for all the nutrients your body needs is the perfect way to ensure your body is healthy and strong. This then raises your energy levels giving you the strength to go about your daily activities and achieve as much as you would wish. Nutrition is also very important therefore if you do a lot of physical activity.
- **Improved Fitness Levels.**
  As explained in Chapter 6, working out goes hand in hand with observing proper nutrition when eating and also when hydrating. You can therefore expect to reach your fitness goals faster and easier if you observe what you take in.
- **Better Body Functioning.**
  By not paying attention to the nutrient value of your food, it is very easy for you to end up missing out on some vital vitamins and minerals which aid your body to function better. Research has shown that fruits and vegetables have very high nutrient content which is crucial to the various body processes from complex ones in the nervous and cardiovascular systems to things as simple as having glowing hair and skin. So if you want to look good, eat better!
- **Better Cardiovascular and Brain Health**
  When it comes to diet-related health complication, these heart and the brain tend to be the most affected body organs. By hydrating properly and eating nutritious meals, you can easily subvert such long—term health problems like hypertension, dementia and Diabetes. Dark fruits and vegetables in particular are best for fighting Alzheimer's disease.

Looking Vibrant and Younger

If you want look amazing, then balanced nutritious meals are the secret. A month of feeding on pure junk will cause your face to break out into a heave of pimples. Eating healthy on the other hand will make your skin appear more youthful and glow. Moreover, having the right nutrients in your body is a sure way to delay the ageing process. Eating right is the key to stopping the wrinkles from kicking in.

Conclusion

Thank you again for downloading this book! If you liked this book please leave a review on amazon. *Link: http://amzn.to/2pKJOEs*

I hope this book was able to help you to understand nutrition better including how to be healthy, what foods are right to eat and what not to eat. Observing nutrition is as simple as that!

The next step now is to do a lifestyle change in terms of your diet. Watch what you eat and ensure you eat the correct amounts of everything. After all, to feel amazing and look amazing, you have to eat right. All the best as you embark on your healthy eating journey!

www.ingramcontent.com/pod-product-compliance
Lightning Source LLC
Chambersburg PA
CBHW072029280526
45788CB00007B/2724